Stomach Exercises Done In Bed

SLATER PRESS
Leo, Indiana

Legal Disclaimer

Before you begin doing these exercises, we strongly recommend that you consult with your physician.

You should be in good physical condition and be able to participate in the exercise before beginning to use these exercises.

The author and publisher or anyone associated with this publication or any associated publications are not licensed medical care providers and represents that it has no expertise in diagnosing, examining, or treating medical conditions of any kind, or in determining the effect of any specific exercise on a medical condition.

You should understand that when participating in any exercise or exercise program, there is the possibility of physical injury. If you engage in this exercise or exercise program, you agree that you do so at your own risk, are voluntarily participating in these activities, assume all risk of injury to yourself, and agree to release and discharge the author and publisher or anyone associated with this publication or any associated publications from any and all claims or causes of action, known or unknown, arising out of the author's or publisher's negligence.

Stomach Exercises Done In Bed

Why Exercise In Bed?

These exercises are provided by Artie McGovern, a physical trainer who worked with such sports professionals as the baseball legend Babe Ruth, world boxing champ Jack Dempsey and gold medalist and multi-sport women's athlete Babe Dickerson among many, many others.

Admit it. We're all inclined towards a sagging gut. But when we bend over and touch the floor with our hands, we only push the internal organs downward when they really need to be pushed upward. By merely lying down you move your internal organs up where they should be and you're able to perform exercises with a fuller range of motion.

That's why these exercises were designed to be done while in bed. And while they mainly focus on the abdominal muscles, they will stimulate all the internal organs to promote circulation and aid elimination of waste.

Why are we stressing exercising the abdominal muscles? Because even sedentary people get some arm and leg exercise during the course of the day. However, the abdomen usually gets no exercise at all.

What proof? Look at your middle. See that fat around the waist and hips? It gets there because that's what's least active. And the abdominal cavity is the only area that is not supported or surrounded by a bony structure; it's entirely sustained by muscle.

Muscle keeps the internal organs in a normal position and when we consider that these organs are among the most important ones we have, you can understand how essential it is to keep them strong.

It's also obvious that well-developed abs aid the digestive, circulatory, and eliminative functions. If these aren't working well your general health will suffer. Honestly, we don't all need those big body-building muscles. What we all DO need is a firm, strong abdominal area.

But these exercises are more than just about the abs. They're about limbering up and toning your entire body. And these exercises are very simple and easy to do. But before you dive in, check them out with your doctor. You can never be too careful.

Start out easy at first and do the ones that you can do. Just don't overdo it. Always bear in mind that the exercises must be done when you are completely relaxed. And above all else, never keep your muscles tense and/or rigid while doing them. Use an easy, flowing motion throughout.

I recommend that you do them first thing in the morning BEFORE you get out of bed. Or if you're bed-ridden, do them any time that is convenient but preferably a couple hours after eating.

To sum up:

- Do all the exercises in bed.
- Don't neglect any of the exercises because they seem too simple.
- Don't overdo it.
- Keep relaxed at all times.
- Exercise regularly. If you don't exercise regularly, you'll accomplish nothing.

Video:
https://www.youtube.com/watch?v=ED2U3VdbDSY

On April 12, 1935, Lou Gehrig and former heavyweight champion Jack Dempsey met at NYC's famous Artie McGovern's Gym.

Artie McGovern

Exercise In Bed

Start out by doing exercises 1-9. They will give you a good workout without over-taxing you. You can do these for a week or two until you feel strong enough to proceed to the next set of exercises.

Only after you feel you are up to it, do exercises 1-9 and then continue with the next exercises up through Exercise 19. It may take you a while to get your body strengthen to complete of these at one time. But you can always do them in up into sets. Do a few, then rest, do a few more, then rest, and so on. There is no set amount you have to do. You are in charge.

When you are up to it you can then progress to doing ALL the exercises in one day or even at one set time. But again, only do what you are able to without over-doing it.

If you find this regimen too strenuous, slow down and take your time. Work your way up gradually. We are not in a race. Just don't overdo it. Let your body tell you what it can and cannot handle.

Exercise 1

1. Lay your back with your shoulders flat on the bed, your hands at your side.
2. With your palms turned downward, exhale slowly and completely.
3. Turn the palms upwards and inhale slowly and deeply while raising your chest and depressing your abdomen.
4. Hold your breath for five seconds.
5. Turn your palms downward and slowly exhale.
6. Relax completely.
7. Repeat six times beginning your count after exhaling.

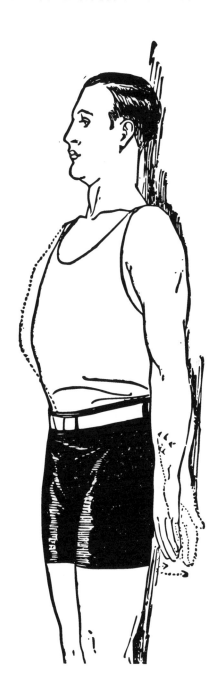

Exercise 2

1. Lay flat on your back and draw your knees up until both feet are flat on the bed as shown in the diagram.
2. Place a weight (a heavy book will do) on your abdomen.
3. Raise the weight by expanding the abdominal muscles and then lower it by relaxing them.
4. Repeat fifteen times counting each time you raise the weight.
5. Rest.
6. Repeat fifteen times more.
7. Rest.
8. Repeat ten more times, making forty in all.

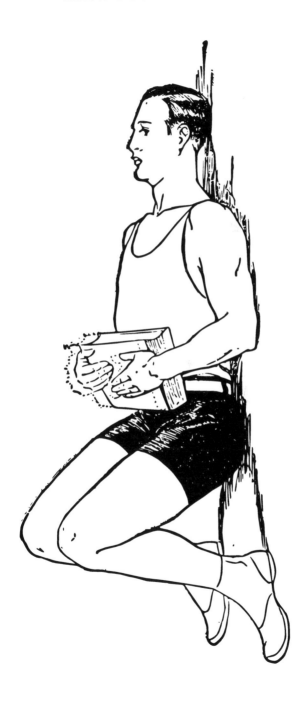

Exercises 3 and 4

1. Lay flat on your back with both hands extended above your head. Place your palms together and raise your left leg upward while bringing your right arm forward towards your leg.
2. Try to touch your toes with your fingers while keeping your leg straight.
3. Return to the starting position without touching the bed with your heel or your hand.
4. Repeat six times counting each time you return to the starting position.
5. Continue but this time switch to your right leg and your left arm. Repeat six times counting each time you return to the starting position.

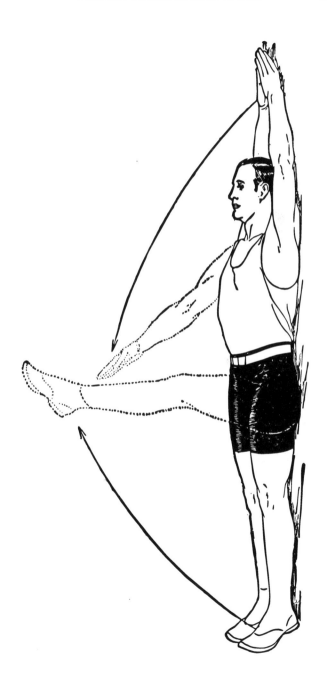

Exercise 5

1. Lay flat on your back with your hips and head down. Extend your arms and legs straight upward.
2. Kick your right leg downward while you bring your left arm up over the head.
3. Alternate with your left leg and your right arm while not touching the bed with either your heels or hands.
4. Repeat six times counting each time the left leg is down.

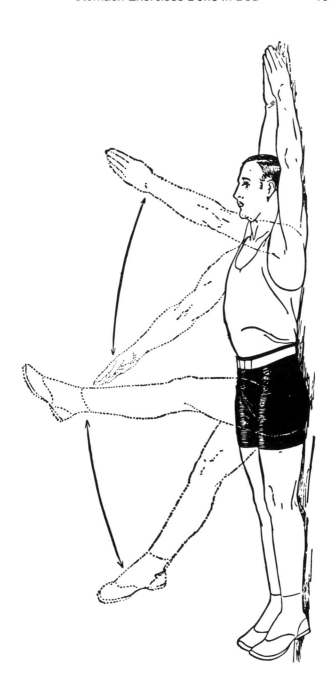

Exercise 6

1. Lay flat on your back with your arms extended above your head.
2. Raise both legs while swinging both your arms upward keeping the outside of the legs and down to the sides while keeping your legs and arms straight.
3. Return to the starting point but without touching the bed.
4. Repeat six times counting each time you return to the starting position.

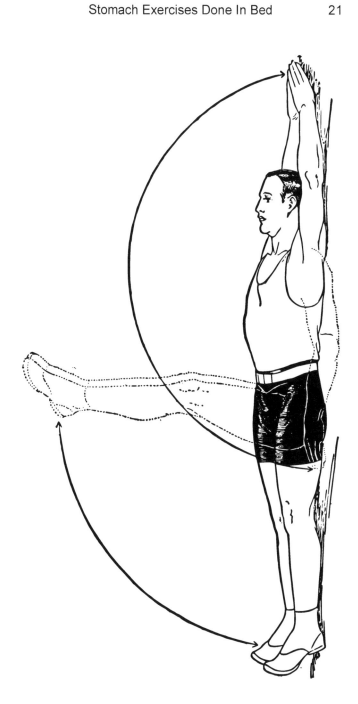

Exercise 7

1. Lay flat on your back and extend both your arms straight above your head while keeping your palms together, as shown in the diagram.
2. Raise your body to a sitting position without bending the knees and try to touch your toes with your finger tips.
3. Repeat six times counting each time you touch the toes.

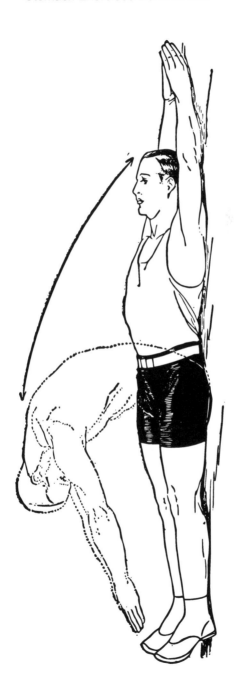

Exercise 8

1. Lay flat on your back and raise both arms and both legs to the upright starting position (see diagram).
2. Keep both arms and legs straight, your palms together and your toes pointed.
3. Spread your arms and your legs outward.
4. Return to the starting position.
5. Repeat six times counting each time your arms and legs come together.

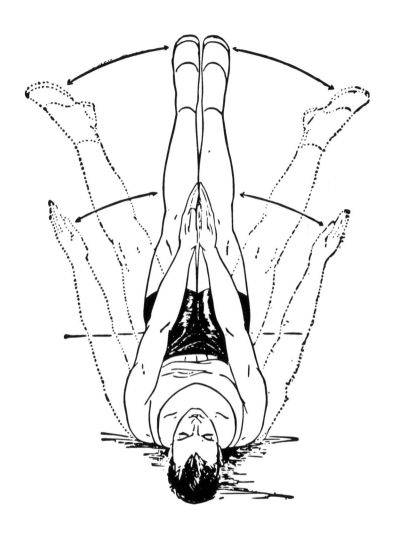

Exercise 9

1. Begin this exercise from the same starting position as in Exercise 8.
2. Cross your arms and your legs, first with the right arm and right leg upper-most.
3. Then do the same thing with your left arm and left leg uppermost.
4. Alternate this movement six times counting each time the right arm and right leg are uppermost.

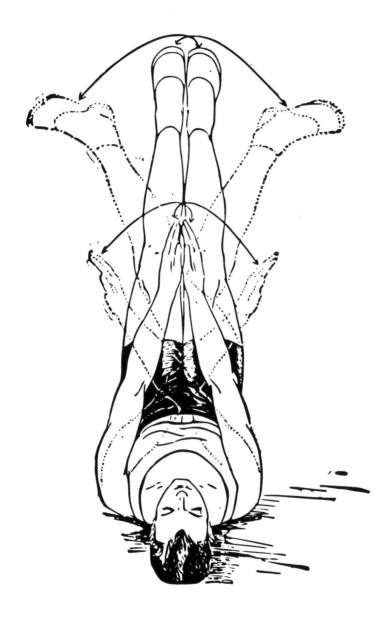

Exercises 10 and 11

1. Lay flat on your back with your hands at your sides.
2. Keeping your legs spread apart, raise the left leg and the right arm upward.
3. Draw a circle with your leg, swinging it out, upward, and in without touching the bed.
4. At the same time draw a circle with your right arm swinging it in, upward, and out.
5. Repeat six times counting each time the circles are completed.
6. Repeat the same movements six times but with the right leg and left arm counting each time the circles are completed.

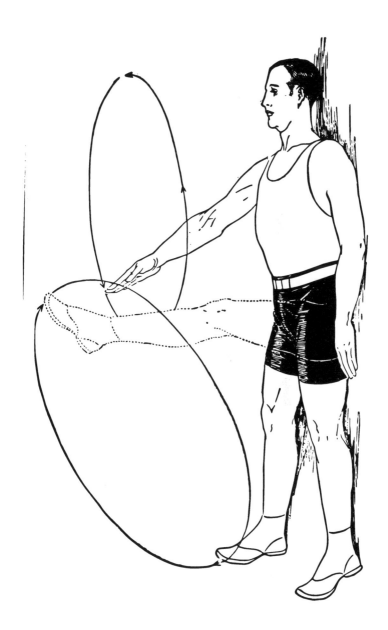

Exercise 12

1. Lay flat on your back with your legs up and at right angles.
2. Your arms should up and straight near the legs.
3. Simultaneously start drawing double circles: circle your left leg and your left arm upward and outward towards the left.
4. Your right leg and your right arm upward and outward to the right.
5. Do not touch the bed with your feet or hands while circling.
6. Repeat six times counting every time you describe a circle.

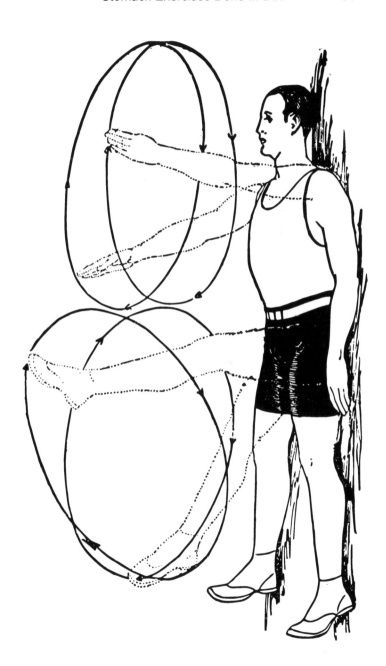

Exercises 13 and 14

1. Lay flat on your back with your hands clasped behind your head.
2. Raise your head and shoulders, drawing your right knee upward while trying to touch your chin or your left shoulder with the knee.
3. Repeat six times counting each time the right leg returns to the starting position.
4. For Exercise 14, do the same movement as before only this time with your left leg.
5. Repeat six times counting each time the leg returns to the starting position.

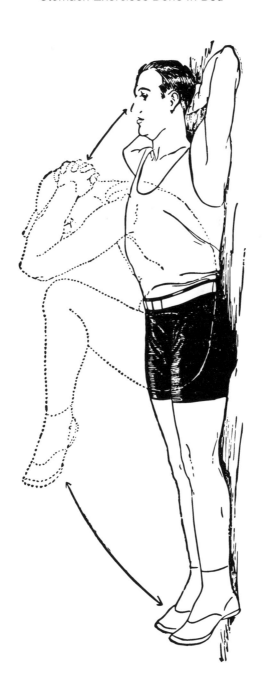

Exercise 15

1. Lay flat on your back with your hands clasped behind your head.
2. Raise both your head and shoulders while drawing up both your knees.
3. At the same time try to touch your chin with your knees.
4. Repeat six times counting each time the legs return to the starting position.

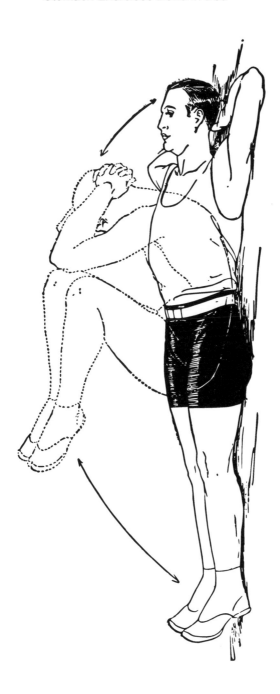

Exercises 16 and 17

1. Lay flat on your back with your hands palms down at your sides.
2. Raise both legs together while keeping the knees stiff and the toes pointed.
3. Circle both legs together to the left making a complete circle without touching the bed.
4. Repeat six times counting each time the legs make a complete circle.
5. Repeat the movement in the opposite direction by circling both legs toward the right six times counting each time the legs make a complete circle.

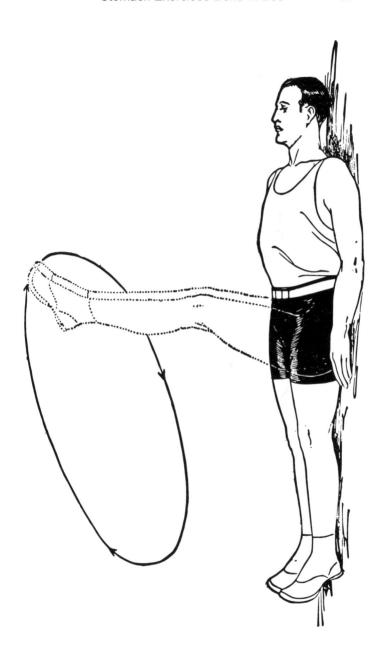

Exercises 18 and 18A

1. Lay on your right side while you place your right hand under your head.
2. Your left hand should be on your left hip.
3. Swing your left leg forward and backward from the hip while keeping the knee stiff and the toes pointed downward.
4. Repeat six times counting each time the leg swings backward.
5. Repeat Exercise 18 but this time lie on your left side and swing your right leg six times counting each time as the leg swings backward.

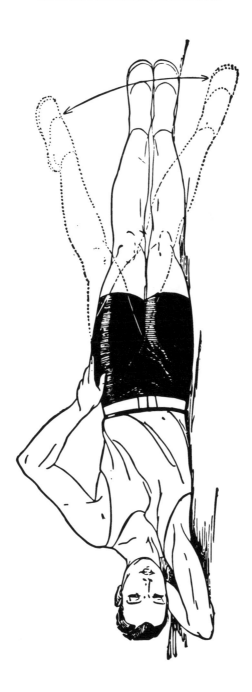

Exercises 19 and 19A

1. Lay on your right side with your right hand under the head and your left hand on your left hip.
2. Draw your left knee up toward your chin while keeping your toes pointed downward.
3. Repeat six times counting each time your leg returns to the straight position.
4. Repeat Exercise 19 using the same movement as before only this time lie on your left side while drawing your right knee up.
5. Repeat six times counting each time your leg returns to the straight position.

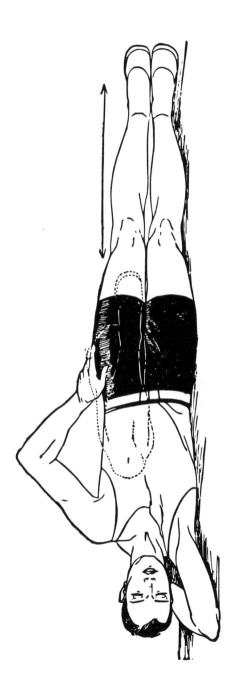

Exercise 20

1. Lay flat on your back while clasping your hands behind your head.
2. Place your feet your toes under a strap or other support to hold the feet securely.
3. Raise your body to a sitting position while bending forward as far as possible.
4. Do not bend the knees in this exercise.
5. Repeat six times counting each time you return to the flat position.

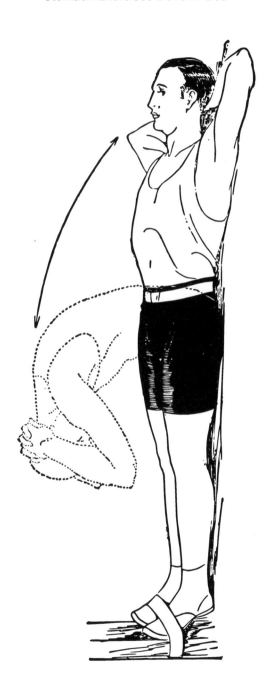

Exercises 21 and 22

1. Sit up on the bed with your toes under a strap or other support and your arms folded across your chest.
2. Make a complete circle with your body by swinging toward the right.
3. Make six complete circles, counting each time you complete a circle.
4. For Exercise 22, circle toward your left six times counting each time you complete a circle.

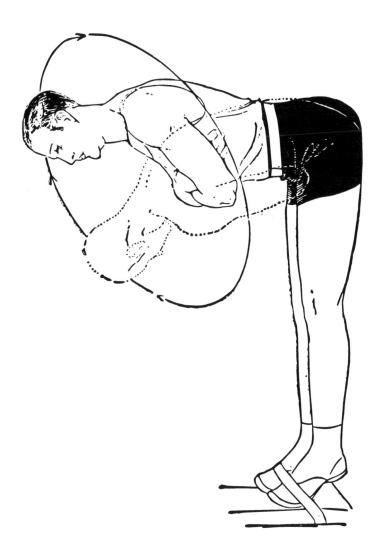

Exercise 23

1. Lay flat on your stomach with your arms folded across your back.
2. Raise your head and shoulders and swing your trunk to the left and then to the right without dropping your head to the bed.
3. Repeat this six times counting each time you swing to the right.

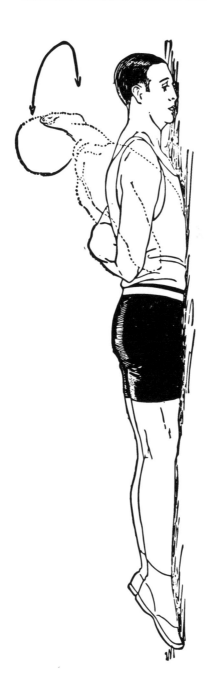

Made in the USA
Columbia, SC
30 January 2023

11264086R00028